LEUKEMIA

PERFECT MEANS FOR TREATING LEUKEMIA

DR. A. RAMOS

Contents

INTRODUCTION

Leukemia is like a rebellious chapter in the intricate history of our blood cells. This specific type of cancer mostly affects blood itself as well as the spongy bone marrow, which is located inside bones and is utilized to make blood cells.

The strange thing is that leukemia results in aberrant blood cell development. Instead of producing fully formed, functional white blood cells, the bone marrow produces abnormal white blood cells known as leukemia cells. Because the defective cells don't carry out their assigned role, the healthy cells are pushed out.

Myeloid or lymphoid leukemia can be classified as either acute or chronic, depending on the specific blood cell that is affected. Possible symptoms include fatigue, bruising or bleeding easily, recurring illnesses, and even weight loss.

Leukemia is like a disruptive character in our health story who needs attention and intervention to turn the tide and bring things back into balance. Treatment options include stem cell transplantation, radiation therapy, and chemotherapy to try to restore equilibrium in the production of red blood cells.

CHAPTER ONE

The Significance of Leukemia

Leukemia is one type of cancer that affects the blood and bone marrow. It involves the abnormal production of white blood cells, which throws off the normal balance of the bloodstream. The bone marrow produces leukemia cells, which are abnormal, immature white blood cells rather than mature, functional white blood cells. These leukemia cells may push out healthy blood cells, which could lead to a number of health issues. Leukemia is classified into different groups according to the kind of blood cell affected (myeloid or lymphoid) and the rate of advancement (acute or chronic). The illness often requires medical intervention, such as chemotherapy, radiation therapy, or stem cell transplantation, to restore a healthy balance of blood cells.

Types of Leukemia

Leukemia comes in different forms, each with unique characteristics. The following are the main categories:

Acute lymphoblastic leukemia (ALL): This rapidly spreading cancer primarily targets lymphoid cells. It generally affects children, though it can also impact adults.

Conversely, Chronic Lymphocytic malignancy (CLL) is a slowly progressing malignancy that primarily attacks mature lymphocytes and is usually found in older adults.

Acute Myeloid Leukemia (AML): A rapidly progressing leukemia affecting myeloid cells. It can affect both adults and children.

Chronic Myeloid Malignancy (CML) is a slowly progressing cancer that affects myeloid cells that is more common in adults.

These classifications are based on the kind of blood cell affected (myeloid or lymphoid) and the rate at which the sickness progresses (acute or chronic). Each type varies in characteristics, treatment options, and prognosis. Developing an effective treatment plan requires determining the precise kind of leukemia.

Acute Lymphoblastic Leukemia (ALL)

The fast-moving, aggressive kind of leukemia known as acute lymphoblastic leukemia (ALL) mostly attacks lymphoid cells, a subgroup of white blood cells. Consider ALL to be the blood cell world's rebel. These days, lymphoid cells are essential to the immune system's function of defending the body against illnesses.

Usually, ALL presents itself quickly, especially in younger people. It is the most common type of leukemia in youngsters, in fact. However, adults can also encounter it. In ALL, immature leukemia cells multiply rapidly, pushing out healthy cells from the bone marrow and bloodstream.

Severe symptoms include bone or joint pain, fatigue, recurring infections, and easy bruising or bleeding can be caused by ALL. The diagnostic procedure involves the use of blood testing, bone marrow biopsies, and occasionally imaging examinations.

But don't be alarmed! Medical superheroes with weapons like chemotherapy, targeted therapy, and stem cell transplantation often step in to help fight ALL. Over the years, ALL research outcomes have significantly improved, especially for children. This improvement can be attributed primarily to medical breakthroughs and superhuman-level treatments.

Features

Among blood cancers, acute lymphoblastic leukemia, or ALL, is distinct because it has the following characteristics:

Fast Onset: ALL progresses swiftly, much like the Usain Bolt kind of leukemia. It typically develops quickly, which means that symptoms start to show up right away.

Lymphoid Cells: The primary constituent of this leukemia is the lymphoid cell. The primary cause of it is the bone marrow's overproduction of immature lymphocytes, which are white blood cells in charge of immune responses.

Childhood Prevalence: Children are more vulnerable to the consequences of ALL. While it does occur in adults, this is the most common type of leukemia in children.

Symptoms: Like warning lights flashing on the body's dashboard, fatigue, recurring infections, easy bruising or bleeding, bone discomfort, and joint pain are common indications of ALL.

Diagnostic Methods: A mix of blood tests, bone marrow biopsies, and imaging techniques may be utilized in the detection of ALL in order to gain a comprehensive image of the body's internal workings.

Treatment Arsenal: Armed with radiation, chemotherapy, targeted therapy, and stem cell transplantation, medical wizards are on the front lines of defense against ALL. The goal is to eliminate the abnormal cells and restore the proper balance of the blood.

Though ALL is a formidable foe, keep in mind that the prognosis for patients has significantly improved because to advances in specialized treatments and medical research.

Risk factors

The illness known as acute lymphoblastic leukemia (ALL) is brought on by both hereditary and environmental factors. The likelihood of this particular blood cancer developing could be increased by the following risk factors:

Age: ALL, like a crafty trickster, frequently preys on children. The most vulnerable age group is children between two and five.

Genetic Factors: It could be inherited. An ALL-ridden sibling increases the danger. Certain genetic disorders, such as Down syndrome, substantially enhance the risk.

Radiation Exposure: Long-term exposure to high radiation levels, whether from environmental factors or medicinal therapies, may raise the risk of developing ALL.

Ironically, there have occasionally been unanticipated outcomes from earlier cancer medicines. Future development of ALL may be made more likely by specific chemotherapy and radiation treatments used to treat other cancers.

A few genetic syndromes: Down syndrome is one of these. Inborn errors of metabolism, such as Li-Fraumeni syndrome and Bloom syndrome, can raise the risk.

Gender: It seems that boys have a somewhat higher chance of developing ALL than females do.

Certain Viral Infections: Exposure to certain viruses, like the Epstein-Barr virus, has been linked to an increased risk of ALL.

Recalling that many individuals with ALL have no known risk factors and that the presence of one or more risk factors does not guarantee the development of ALL is critical. Current research is being conducted to determine how environment and genetics combine to form the superhero origin story of ALL.

Symptoms and indicators

The symptoms of acute lymphoblastic leukemia (ALL) can be very diverse. If you believe ALL is plotting something bad, keep an eye out for these signs:

Fatigue: After a marathon-length run, try to envision hardly being able to move. Weakness and extreme weariness are possible outcomes of ALL.

Frequently Getting Infections: Your body is not functioning at its best. Extended healing periods, repeated infections, and heightened vulnerability to infections may serve as warning signs for ALL.

Simple Bleeding or Bruising: ALL lowers blood platelet counts by disrupting the normal production of red blood cells. This could result in easy bruising, bleeding gums, or nosebleeds.

Bone and Joint Pain: Bone or joint pain may be caused by leukemia cells invading the bone marrow.

Pale Skin: Low amounts of healthy red blood cells, or anemia, can result in pale skin.

Swollen lymph nodes: When aberrant lymphocytes gather in the lymph nodes, the nodes may swell.

Unexplained Weight Loss: Allergic reactions may affect appetite and metabolism, leading to unexplained weight loss.

Fever: When leukemia cells obstruct the body's ability to combat infections, fever can happen without apparent explanation.

If you notice that these symptoms are persisting or are growing worse, you should consult a healthcare professional immediately. Early detection and management can significantly improve outcomes in the fight against ALL.

Medical professionals must employ a detective-like method to diagnose ALL, an elusive disease. The vital steps to find this blood malignancy are as follows:

Clinical Evaluation: A thorough examination of your prior medical records and a discussion of your symptoms are the first steps in the process. Prepare to provide your health information with the medical investigator.

Blood Tests: The abnormal levels of white blood cells, red blood cells, and platelets that can be observed in a blood test are a crucial clue in the ALL investigation.

The real investigation begins with the biopsy and bone marrow aspiration. A tiny sample of bone marrow is taken from the hip bone using a needle. Next, this sample is examined under a microscope to check for leukemia cells.

A spinal tap, sometimes referred to as a lumbar puncture, entails drawing cerebrospinal fluid from the spinal canal.

CHAPTER TWO

It helps determine whether the central nervous system has been colonized by leukemia cells.

Imaging studies: X-rays, CT scans, or MRIs may be performed to get an interior picture and look for any signs of leukemia infiltration.

Cytogenetic analysis: The chromosomes of the leukemia cells are examined in this detailed analysis. Certain genetic changes can help identify the kind of leukemia and provide important information about therapy options.

Once the medical team has all of these jigsaw pieces assembled, they will be able to construct a comprehensive diagnosis of ALL. Early discovery is crucial in the fight against this blood cancer, which is spreading quickly, as it sets the stage for timely and effective therapies.

Treatment options

To combat Acute Lymphoblastic Leukemia (ALL), a variety of pharmacological medications are required. Among the principal players in the treatment are the following:

Chemotherapy is the front-line warrior. Strong drugs are used to stop leukemia cells from growing or to completely eradicate them. Chemotherapy can be administered via injection into the spinal fluid, orally, or intravenously.

Think of focused therapy as the squad that delivers accurate hits. Targeted drugs are designed to specifically target certain substances that contribute to the growth of leukemia cells while minimizing damage to healthy cells.

Radiation therapy: High-energy radiation is occasionally used to target and kill leukemia cells. It is common practice to prepare for a stem cell transplant by doing this.

Transplanting stem cells: The best possible help. Stem cells from an allogeneic donor or the patient themselves are transplanted to replace the damaged bone marrow with healthy cells. This is often an essential part of treatment, especially when there is a substantial risk involved.

Immunotherapy: This employs the body's own defenses against the enemy. Immunotherapy drugs help the immune system identify leukemia cells and destroy them more effectively.

Just as crucial as the heavy guns is supportive care. This include managing symptoms, treating and preventing infections, and giving platelet infusions or blood transfusions when necessary.

When developing the treatment plan, considerations such as the patient's age, other personal characteristics, and the specifics of their leukemia are often taken into account. It's a dynamic, ever-evolving method where doctors review and adjust the plan on a regular basis based on treatment results. The goal? To send EVERYONE packing and restore harmony to the blood cell kingdom.

Acute Myeloid Leukemia (AML)

Acute myeloid leukemia (AML) is comparable to the rebel commander in the blood cell story. Aggressive and fast-moving, this leukemia upends everything in its path.

Here's the synopsis:

Myeloid cells are the target of AML; these cells are important in the production of certain types of white blood cells, red blood cells, and platelets.

Quick Onset: AML, like its acute lymphoblastic brother, is all about speed. Its characteristic is the rapid proliferation of aberrant and immature myeloid cells.

Age Factor: AML usually appears later in life and is more common in the elderly. However, it can affect individuals of all ages, including children.

Symptoms: AML symptoms resemble warning indicators in the body. Weariness, recurring infections, easy bruising or bleeding, and soreness in the bones are common symptoms.

Blood, bone marrow aspiration and biopsy, and occasionally genetic testing are part of the diagnosis process for acute myeloid leukemia (AML) in order to provide a whole picture.

Odyssey of Treatment: Following a diagnosis of AML, a treatment plan is often initiated. Chemotherapy is an essential part of the strategy to replace bad bone marrow with healthy cells; in certain cases, a stem cell transplant may also be part of the approach.

Though AML remains a formidable opponent, advancements in medical science and targeted treatments are enhancing outcomes and offering optimism in the struggle against this swiftly advancing and highly aggressive form of leukemia.

Features

Acute Myeloid Leukemia (AML) is distinguished by a special confluence of characteristics that contribute to its position within the intricate narrative of blood cancers:

Myeloid Cell Takeover: Myeloid cells, the main target of AML, are essential for the synthesis of red blood cells, platelets, and certain forms of white blood cells.

Rapid Growth: The rapid proliferation of immature and abnormal myeloid cells, which impairs normal blood cell production, is a hallmark of acute myeloid leukemia (AML). It resembles a bone marrow wildfire.

Age Affiliation: Although AML can affect a person at any age, it usually choose to manifest itself later in life. Older people are more prone to encounter it, and the likelihood increases with age.

AML does not present with modest symptoms. It requires medical attention to manage its symptoms, which include soreness in the bones, easy bruising or bleeding, fatigue, and recurring infections.

AML is diagnosed through a series of procedures that include bone marrow aspiration and biopsy, blood tests, and sometimes genetic testing. This comprehensive approach helps to expose the features of the leukemia.

Treatment Strategies: Chemotherapy is the cornerstone of the AML defense. The goal is to eliminate the abnormal cells so that the bone marrow can produce red blood cells that are healthy again. In certain cases, a stem cell transplant may be an option.

Genetic Diversity: There isn't just one approach to treating AML. Variations in the genetic makeup of leukemia cells affect the prognosis and treatment options.

Prognostic Factors: The patient's age, the specific genetic abnormalities they have, and how well they respond to treatment are all important factors that affect the prognosis for AML. Targeted and tailored methods are essential due to this complexity.

These characteristics are similar to the AML language, allowing medical professionals to successfully navigate the remission road and tailor treatment approaches.

Many genetic and environmental variables might increase an individual's risk of acquiring acute myeloid leukemia (AML), a particular kind of blood cancer. The following are some important risk factors:

Age: Later life periods are often preferred by AML. The probability increases with age, and those who are older have a higher chance of receiving a diagnosis.

It's interesting to note that previous cancer therapy may occasionally lead to the development of AML. Certain chemotherapy drugs and radiation therapies, especially those used to treat conditions like lymphoma or breast cancer, may raise the risk.

Genetic Syndromes: Several hereditary syndromes, such as Li-Fraumeni syndrome or Fanconi anemia, as well as Down syndrome are associated with an elevated risk of AML.

Radiation Exposure: Prolonged exposure to high radiation levels can be hazardous, whether it's from workplace exposure or radiation therapy for medical conditions.

Different Chemical Exposures: Research has shown a connection between increased risk and exposure to a number of chemicals, such as benzene, which is present in some industrial settings, and tobacco smoke.

Smoking: It is believed that smoking cigarettes raises the risk of AML in relation to tobacco smoke.

Gender: AML shows a slight predilection toward men over women.

Blood disorders: Individuals with pre-existing blood disorders, such as myelodysplastic syndromes (MDS), are at a higher risk.

It is important to keep in mind that having one or more risk factors does not guarantee the development of AML, and many individuals who receive an AML diagnosis do not have any known risk factors. Studies on the interplay of these factors in the complex tale of leukemia are still in progress.

Symptoms and indicators

AML is characterized by a variety of symptoms that point to a disruption in the normal functioning of red blood cells. Keep an eye out for any of the following potential warning signs:

Fatigue: AML can make you feel as though you've run a marathon, even with no physical effort.

Frequently Become Infected: AML attacks healthy white blood cells, lowering immunity and making you more susceptible to infections.

Easy Bruising or Bleeding: AML may result in nosebleeds, bleeding gums, or easy bruising since it decreases platelet formation.

Leukemia cells have the capacity to penetrate the bone marrow and induce joint and bone discomfort.

Pale Skin: A shortage of healthy red blood cells might result in fatigue and pallor.

Breathlessness: As anemia is a common side effect of AML, shortness of breath may be the result of reduced oxygen-carrying ability.

Unexplained Weight Loss: AML may have an impact on appetite and metabolism, which could result in unexplained weight loss.

Fever: Leukemia cells have the potential to impair the body's defenses against infections, leading to fevers that flare up frequently and seemingly out of the blue.

If you notice that these symptoms are persisting or are growing worse, you should consult a healthcare professional immediately. An early diagnosis and treatment start can have a significant impact on the outcome of the fight against AML.

Recognition

The first stage in diagnosing acute myeloid leukemia (AML), which is confirmed by a battery of medical examinations and tests, is finding abnormal myeloid cells in the bone marrow and blood. An overview of the diagnostic process is provided below:

Clinical Evaluation: At the beginning of the journey, your medical history is carefully reviewed, taking into account any symptoms you may be experiencing. Your healthcare professional will also do a physical examination.

Blood Tests: A simple blood sample can give important clues. AML is commonly linked to abnormally high levels of platelets, red blood cells, and white blood cells.

Bone marrow aspiration and biopsy: This is a crucial step. A tiny sample of bone marrow is taken from the hip bone using a needle. Next, the sample is examined under a microscope to check for leukemia cells. This provides information about the type of leukemia, its genetic composition, and the extent of bone marrow involvement.

The chromosomes of leukemia cells are examined as part of the cytogenetic analysis process. Certain genetic changes can affect treatment options and prognosis.

Flow Cytometry: By analyzing the characteristics of the cells, this technique aids in the identification of abnormal leukemia cells in the blood or bone marrow.

Immunophenotyping: This method helps determine the kind of leukemia by examining the proteins on the surface of cells.

Lumbar Puncture (Spinal Tap): Under some conditions, a lumbar puncture may be required to obtain a sample of cerebrospinal fluid from the spinal canal. This makes it easier to determine whether the central nervous system has been colonized by leukemia cells.

Imaging studies: X-rays, CT scans, or MRIs may be carried out to ascertain whether leukemia cells have spread to other organs or tissues.

By putting these diagnostic pieces together, doctors may determine the specific type of leukemia, assess how severe the disease is, and create a treatment plan that is appropriate and tailored to the particulars of acute myeloid leukemia. Having an accurate and timely diagnosis is essential to initiating timely and effective therapy.

To treat Acute Myeloid Leukemia (AML), which is an aggressive disease, many treatment strategies are required. Crucial players in the battle against this aggressive blood malignancy are the following people:

When it comes to treating AML, chemotherapy is the clear heavyweight champion. Strong drugs are used to either destroy leukemia cells or stop their growth. Induction chemotherapy is the initial stage of treatment, with the goal of inducing remission. In order to prevent recurrence, consolidation and maintenance therapy are thereafter given.

Transplanting stem cells is similar to a biological reboot. Stem cells from an allogeneic donor or the patient themselves are transplanted to replace the damaged bone marrow with healthy cells. This is often considered for individuals with high-risk AML.

Targeted treatment epitomizes precision medicine at its best. Targeted drugs are designed to specifically target certain substances that contribute to the growth of leukemia cells while minimizing damage to healthy cells.

Clinical Trials: Participating in clinical trials can advance leukemia research and provide participants with access to cutting-edge medicines, as AML treatment is still an evolving field.

Just as crucial as the heavy guns is supportive care. This include managing symptoms, treating and preventing infections, and giving platelet infusions or blood transfusions when necessary.

Differentiation Therapy: Using a technique known as differentiation therapy, a few more modern medications help leukemia cells develop into healthy red blood cells.

Immunotherapy: Using the body's immune system to target and eradicate leukemia cells. Monoclonal antibodies, among other immunotherapy-related drugs, are being studied for the treatment of AML.

Radiation therapy: One method for treating leukemia cells in specific areas is targeted radiation therapy.

When developing the treatment plan, considerations such as the patient's age, other personal characteristics, and the specifics of their leukemia are often taken into account. It's a dynamic, ever-evolving method where doctors review and adjust the plan on a regular basis based on treatment results. The goal? in order to end AML and provide the groundwork for a viable future free of leukemia.

Chronic Lymphocytic Leukemia (CLL)

The wise old man of leukemias, Chronic Lymphocytic Leukemia (CLL), is a slow-growing, mostly indolent form that primarily targets lymphocytes, a specific kind of white blood cell.

Let's get more detailed now:

Lymphocytic Domination: Lymphocytes, a part of the immune system, are the main target of CLL. These cells overproliferate in CLL, yet they are often ineffective.

Chronic Nature: As its name suggests, CLL is a chronic illness, which means that it advances slowly. It is often found in elderly people, and many may not have any symptoms for some time.

Age Association: Older people tend to attract CLL more. It is more common in adults, especially in those over 60.

Symptoms: CLL can produce symptoms even if they appear gradually. Typical symptoms include fatigue, enlarged lymph nodes, unintentional weight loss, and recurring infections.

Diagnosis Adventure: Diagnosing CLL involves a number of procedures, including imaging studies, bone marrow biopsies, and blood testing. An increase in abnormal lymphocyte counts in the blood is the defining finding.

Watch and Wait: Due to the slow progression of CLL, not all patients require immediate initiation of medication. In rare cases, a "watch and wait" approach may be employed, involving continuous monitoring until the condition deteriorates.

Treatment Options: When required, a combination of immunotherapy, chemotherapy, and targeted therapy may be employed. The patient's health and the stage of the disease are among the many factors that go into the choice.

Prognosis: Many CLL patients live for years, despite the fact that the disease is typically considered incurable. The prognosis varies widely, and the disease's course is uncertain.

Understanding CLL is similar to studying the story of a wise friend and patient in the complex world of blood cancers. The complexities of this condition necessitate careful consideration and a personalized treatment strategy, even though it may not necessarily require immediate attention.

Features

Chronic lymphocytic leukemia (CLL) is characterized by a distinct set of traits that define its nature and behavior within the intricate area of blood cancers:

Overproduction of Lymphocytes: The development of CLL depends primarily on B cells. These cells multiply uncontrolled, but they also typically exhibit abnormal behavior.

Compared to its acute brethren, CLL is an indolent leukemia that grows more slowly. It often progresses slowly, and many people may go for a long period without experiencing any symptoms at all.

Age Affiliation: Later life periods are where CLL is most prevalent. It is more common to diagnose adults, especially those over 60.

Early Stages: In its asymptomatic state, CLL may not even produce any symptoms, keeping patients in the dark about the disease. It is often discovered by accident during routine blood tests.

Common Symptoms: These could include exhaustion, enlarged lymph nodes, unintentional weight loss, recurring infections, and a feeling of fullness or soreness behind the ribs.

"Watch and Wait" strategy: Not every CLL patient needs treatment immediately soon. In certain cases, a "watch and wait" or "watch and worry" approach may be employed, entailing continuous monitoring until the condition deteriorates.

The Diagnosis Adventure: Blood tests reveal a greater number of abnormal cells in the CLL diagnosis. A bone marrow sample and imaging studies are typically required for a confirmation.

Plans for Treatment: When therapy is necessary, immunotherapy, chemotherapy, targeted therapy, or a combination of these may be used. The patient's condition and the stage of the disease are among the many factors that go into the choice.

Prognosis Variability: Although there are wide variations in the prognosis of CLL, the disease is usually regarded as incurable. While some people may live longer and see no change in their quality of life, others may follow a more aggressive path.

Medical professionals can better manage the unique journeys of CLL patients and tailor treatment plans to fit the specific needs and characteristics of the illness by being aware of these factors.

CHAPTER THREE

Risk factors

While chronic lymphoblastic leukemia (CLL) is a blood cancer that progresses slowly, some factors may increase the risk of developing it. A few potential risk factors are as follows:

Age: Like a quiet spouse, the frequency of CLL rises with age. It is often found in older adults, with an increasing risk beyond the age of 60.

Genes: Ancestral history could be important. If you have a parent or sibling in your immediate family who has had CLL, your risk may be somewhat elevated.

Gender: People with CLL typically identify as men. Men are more prone than women to get CLL.

Ethnicity: People of European descent usually have higher rates of CLL, while the prevalence varies depending on the ethnic group.

Exposure to Particular Chemicals: Research has linked the usage of pesticides and herbicides during work to an increased risk of developing chronic lymphocytic leukemia (CLL). However, the evidence is not conclusive.

Exposure to Agent Orange: There may be a modest increase in risk for Vietnam War veterans who were exposed to the pesticide Agent Orange.

Family History of Other Blood Cancers: Multiple myeloma and non-Hodgkin lymphoma, while unrelated blood cancers, might influence a person's risk of acquiring CLL.

It's important to keep in mind that many CLL patients have no known risk factors, and that having one or more of these risk factors does not guarantee that CLL will manifest. The complex interactions between genetic and environmental factors that influence the risk of leukemia are still being studied.

Symptoms and indicators

Chronic lymphocytic leukemia (CLL) is a slow-growing leukemia, therefore symptoms may not always be noticeable at first. In actuality, some individuals may go for extended periods of time without displaying any symptoms. However, when symptoms do arise, they could include:

Weakness: Frequently a companion in numerous chronic conditions, fatigue in CLL can be persistent and impede daily activities.

Enlarged Lymph Nodes: CLL often leads to an excess of lymphocytes that are not normal, which makes the lymph nodes grow.

Unintentional Weight Loss: Individuals with CLL may unintentionally lose weight without any apparent cause.

Recurrent Infections: Because the aberrant cells in CLL are not operating normally, the immune system may be weakened and more susceptible to infections.

Night Sweats: Those who have chronic lymphoblastic leukemia (CLL) may experience painful night sweats that disrupt their sleep.

Abdominal Discomfort: An enlarged spleen or liver is a common symptom of CLL and can cause discomfort or a sense of fullness in the abdomen.

Easy Bleeding or Bruising: Because CLL may inhibit the normal production of platelets, bleeding or bruising may be simpler to handle.

Painless Lumps: Unlike infections that may result in painful lymph nodes, swollen lymph nodes in CLL usually do not cause any discomfort.

Notably, there might be notable individual differences in the duration and severity of symptoms. Additionally, some CLL patients may continue for a long period without exhibiting any symptoms, and routine blood testing may accidentally reveal their illness. If your symptoms are getting worse or are reoccurring, see a healthcare professional for a thorough evaluation and diagnosis.

Recognition

Many steps need to be done in order to interpret the moderate signs of Chronic Lymphocytic Leukemia (CLL), a slow-growing blood cancer.

An overview of the diagnostic process is provided below:

Clinical Evaluation: A thorough history of your previous health and a discussion of any symptoms you may be experiencing are the first steps in the procedure. Your healthcare provider will check your body for physical symptoms such swollen lymph nodes, liver, or spleen.

Blood Tests: Relevant information can be obtained from a simple blood sample. In patients with CLL, a complete blood count (CBC) may reveal a higher than normal lymphocyte count. You may need more blood tests to assess the overall health of your blood and organs.

Flow Cytometry: By examining the characteristics of the cells in a sample, this specialized technique helps identify abnormal lymphocytes. It is a vital tool for CLL diagnosis.

Aspiration and Bone Marrow Biopsy: If CLL is suspected, a small sample of bone marrow from the hip bone may be extracted using a needle. After that, the overall health of the bone marrow and the presence of leukemia cells are assessed by microscopically examining this sample.

Immunophenotyping: This method looks at the proteins on the surface of cells to help determine the kind of leukemia and confirm that CLL is present.

Cytogenetic analysis: This technique examines the chromosomes in the leukemia cells to reveal information on the genetic composition of CLL.

Imaging studies: Imaging tests such as CT scans may occasionally be used to measure the size of the liver, spleen, or lymph nodes.

Once these jigsaw pieces are put together, your healthcare team will be able to assess the disease's stage, validate the CLL diagnosis, and develop a monitoring or treatment strategy. Not every patient has to begin therapy immediately away because CLL advances slowly; in some cases, a watch-and-wait approach may be employed. Early and accurate diagnosis is key to timely and tailored treatment of this chronic blood cancer.

Care must be taken when treating Chronic Lymphocytic Leukemia (CLL) in order to maintain quality of life. Treatment decisions are influenced by several factors, such as the stage of the disease, the patient's overall health, and the presence of symptoms. Typical options for treating CLL include the following:

Watch and Wait (Observation): This tactic may be employed in some circumstances, especially if the illness is still in its early stages and there are no symptoms. Regular monitoring helps health care providers avoid unnecessary treatments and take appropriate action when needed.

Chemotherapy: Using standard chemotherapy drugs, leukemia cells can be eliminated or their growth inhibited. Modern targeted therapies are often selected due to their higher efficacy and decreased toxicity, even while older medications are still available.

Targeted therapy: To lessen damage to healthy cells, these drugs are designed to specifically target specific molecules that are necessary for the growth of CLL cells. Three examples of popular targeted medications are inhibitors of BTK, PI3K, and BCL-2.

Immunotherapy: The immune system's ability to identify and eradicate leukemia cells can be enhanced by the use of monoclonal antibodies, such as rituximab and obinutuzumab.

Allogeneic stem cell transplantation: A suitable donor stem cell transplant may be an option for a patient with more aggressive or relapsed CLL. Those who get this significant surgery are frequently younger and in better condition.

Clinical Trials: Enrolling in clinical trials can provide access to novel medications and further CLL research. These clinical trials assess new therapies or combinations of therapies.

conjunction Therapies: A variety of drugs may be administered in conjunction for a more comprehensive and effective therapy. This can involve the combination of many pharmaceutical classes, targeted therapies, or immunotherapy.

Supportive Care: Maintaining overall health and managing symptoms are crucial aspects of treating CLL. This may mean managing infections, addressing anemia, and providing supportive care as needed.

Treatment options are highly individualized, and the patient's overall health, genetics, and illness stage all play a role in the therapy selection process. The field of CLL research is still developing, which will improve treatment options and prognoses for people who have this chronic leukemia.

Chronic Myeloid Leukemia (CML)

When it comes to leukemias, Chronic Myeloid Leukemia (CML) is similar to the Painstaking

Conductor; it is a slow-growing, chronic form of the disease marked by an excess of myeloid cells, a particular kind of white blood cell. The Philadelphia chromosome is one distinct genetic marker linked to CML.

Let's examine more closely:

Overproduction of Myeloid Cells: Because myeloid cells are necessary for the production of platelets, red blood cells, and several types of white blood cells, they are the focus of chronic myeloid leukemia (CML).

The Blast Phase, Accelerated Phase, and Chronic Phase are the three stages that CML typically progresses through. During the chronic phase, leukemia cells develop slowly and may not exhibit any symptoms. It can proceed to the faster phase and, in the end, the more violent blast phase if nothing is done.

Philadelphia Chromosome: This genetic abnormality is one of the key features of CML. The abnormal BCR-ABL1 gene is the product of a genetic material translocation that takes place between chromosomes 9 and 22. This fusion gene produces a protein that induces the overproduction of myeloid cells.

Age Distribution: Adult diagnoses of CML are more common, with a median age of roughly 60, despite the fact that the disease can hit anyone at any age.

Symptoms: During the chronic phase, people with CML may not initially show any symptoms. Symptoms including fatigue, weight loss, abdominal pain, and an enlarged spleen may develop as the disease progresses.

Diagnosis Using Blood and Bone Marrow Tests: Blood tests reveal an elevated white blood cell count, and genetic testing verifies the existence of the Philadelphia chromosome. The aspiration and biopsy of bone marrow are often performed to assess the extent of leukemia involvement.

Tyrosine kinase inhibitors (TKIs): One of these specific drugs is the primary treatment for chronic myeloid leukemia (CML). They work by blocking the action of the abnormal BCR-ABL1 protein, which helps to control the excess myeloid cell population. Imatinib, dasatinib, and nilotinib are examples of TKIs.

Stem Cell Transplant: For some individuals, especially those who are in the blast phase or who don't respond well to TKIs, a stem cell transplant may be an option. This means grafting healthy stem cells into the bone marrow that has been damaged.

With the use of customized medications like TKIs, many individuals with CML are able to enjoy normal, productive lives. Effective disease management mostly involves regular monitoring and a customized treatment strategy.

Features

The behavior of chronic myeloid leukemia (CML) in the intricate realm of blood malignancies is characterized by the following distinctive features:

Overproduction of Myeloid Cells: The blood contains an excess of myeloid cells, such as platelets and granulocytes, as a result of Chronic Myeloid Leukemia (CML).

The Philadelphia Chromosome is similar to the unique genetic abnormality that causes chronic myeloid leukemia. The Philadelphia chromosome is the consequence of a translocation between chromosomes 9 and 22 that generates the BCR-ABL1 fusion gene. This gene produces a protein that promotes the uncontrolled growth of myeloid cells.

CHAPTER FOUR

Three Phases: CML usually progresses through three primary stages. Cells with leukemia proliferate gradually and continuously throughout the chronic stage. If therapy is not obtained, it can advance to the accelerated phase and eventually the more severe blast phase, which is comparable to acute leukemia.

Age Distribution: Adult diagnoses of CML are more common, with middle-aged and older individuals having the highest prevalence, despite the fact that the disease can affect anyone at any age.

Chronic Phase Symptoms: During the chronic phase, people with CML may not initially show any symptoms. As the illness progresses, symptoms like fatigue, weight loss, stomach discomfort, and an enlarged spleen may manifest.

Peripheral Blood and Bone Marrow Involvement: Elevated white blood cell counts are often indicated by elevated granulocyte counts in blood tests. Because bone marrow aspiration and biopsy demonstrate the existence of leukemia cells and the unique Philadelphia chromosome, they are utilized to confirm the diagnosis.

The first line of treatment for CML is tyrosine kinase inhibitors, or TKIs. TKIs, such as dasatinib, imatinib, and nilotinib, work by blocking the abnormal BCR-ABL1 protein from doing its job, which helps control the growth of leukemia cells.

Stem Cell Transplant: For some individuals, especially those who are in the blast phase or who don't respond well to TKIs, a stem cell transplant may be an option. This means grafting healthy stem cells into the bone marrow that has been damaged.

Medical professionals can better manage the unique journeys of CML patients and tailor treatment plans to fit the unique needs and characteristics of the illness at different phases if they are aware of these attributes. Many patients may now manage CML as a chronic illness thanks to early detection and targeted therapy.

When chronic myeloid leukemia (CML) first appears, a clear explanation is frequently absent, and certain risk factors are not always understood. However, a few factors may be associated with an increased chance of developing CML:

Age: Adult diagnoses of CML are more common, with a median age of roughly 60, however the disease can hit anyone at any age. The risk usually increases with age.

Radiation Exposure: Prolonged high-dose ionizing radiation exposure, such as that received during various medical operations or at work, has been linked to an increased risk of chronic myeloid leukemia.

Genetic Factors: There may be some genetic commonality even though CML is not typically inherited. However, most cases of CML are unconnected to a family history of the disease.

Gender: The risk of developing CML is slightly higher in men than in women.

Prior Chemotherapy or Radiation Therapy: Individuals with a history of particular cancer treatments, particularly those involving alkylating medications or radiation therapy, may be somewhat more likely to develop CML. Still, the risk in its whole is negligible.

Specific Genetic Abnormalities: While most CML cases are associated with the Philadelphia chromosome (BCR-ABL1 fusion gene), other genetic abnormalities are occasionally found to be involved as well.

It's important to keep in mind that CML usually occurs seldom and that most affected individuals are not at risk for the disease. Moreover, the total probability of getting CML is very low.

If you are worried about your chance of developing CML or any other health condition, it is best to speak with your healthcare provider. Regular monitoring and physicals can also aid in the early detection of these issues.

Chronic myeloid leukemia (CML) usually develops slowly in the early stages and may not show any symptoms. However, when the illness worsens, symptoms may become more apparent. Common indications of CML include:

Fatigue: Persistent, inexplicable fatigue is one of the most common signs of CML. It might have an impact on daily activities and quality of life.

Discomfort in the abdomen: Splenomegaly, or an enlarged spleen, and less commonly, liver enlargement, can cause pain or a sensation of fullness in the abdomen.

Inadvertent Weight Loss: Individuals with CML may have weight loss without realizing it. This is often the consequence of a combination of factors, such as the leukemia cells consuming more energy and decreasing appetite.

Nighttime excessive sweating that is unrelated to temperature or other environmental factors may indicate chronic myeloid leukemia.

Enlarged Lymph Nodes: CML can cause lymph node enlargement, albeit this is less common than in other types of leukemia.

Joint or Bone Pain: Some CML patients may experience joint or bone pain.

Bruising and Bleeding: CML can lead to nosebleeds, bleeding gums, and easy bruising due to its ability to disrupt platelet synthesis.

Frequently Occurring Infections: White blood cell activity may be compromised by CML, increasing the risk of infection.

It's important to keep in mind that these symptoms can arise from a variety of different medical conditions and are not exclusive to CML. Additionally, many patients with CML may not exhibit any symptoms at all during the chronic stage, and the disease may inadvertently be discovered through routine blood tests.

If your symptoms are getting worse or are becoming more persistent, or if you believe you may have CML, you should consult a healthcare professional for a thorough evaluation and diagnosis. Early detection and therapy can have a significant impact on the prognosis for CML patients.

Recognition

Diagnosing chronic myeloid leukemia (CML) involves several steps, such as pinpointing the specific characteristics of the disease and verifying the presence of leukemia cells. An overview of the diagnostic process is provided below:

Clinical Evaluation: At the beginning of the journey, your medical history is carefully reviewed, taking into account any symptoms you may be experiencing. Your healthcare provider will check for signs such an enlarged liver or spleen during a physical examination.

Complete Blood Count (CBC): Typically, a simple blood test is the first step. One potential side effect of CML is an increase in the number of white blood cells, particularly granulocytes. Other blood parameters, such as hemoglobin and platelet counts, can also be assessed.

Perimeter Blood Smear: A blood smear is examined under a microscope to check for abnormal cells, such as blasts or immature granulocytes.

Aspiration and Biopsy of Bone Marrow: Should CML be suspected, a small sample of bone marrow from the hip bone may be extracted using a needle. Subsequently, this sample is examined under a microscope to ascertain the number and characteristics of distinct blood cells. The presence of the Philadelphia chromosome, a genetic hallmark of CML, can often be verified by cytogenetic analysis performed on the bone marrow cells.

Genetic Testing: Molecular methods like as fluorescence in situ hybridization (FISH) and polymerase chain reaction (PCR) may be employed to determine the presence of the BCR-ABL1 fusion gene that is particular to CML.

Imaging studies: Imaging investigations such as CT or ultrasound scans may occasionally be performed to measure the size of the liver or spleen.

Once these diagnostic components are obtained, your healthcare team will be able to confirm the diagnosis of CML, assess the disease's phase (chronic, accelerated, or blast phase), and choose the optimal course of therapy. An accurate and timely diagnosis is essential for improving the prognosis of CML patients and initiating timely therapy.

Treatment options

The therapy of Chronic Myeloid Leukemia (CML) has advanced significantly, making this once-difficult condition today very manageable. The primary goal of treatment is to target the abnormal BCR-ABL1 protein, which is connected to the Philadelphia chromosome and induces the overproduction of myeloid cells. Important options for CML therapy include the following:

Tyrosine kinase Inhibitors (TKIs): This family of targeted drugs is the cornerstone of treatment for CML. They work by blocking the action of the mutated BCR-ABL1 protein. Typical TKIs include:

1. Imatinib
2. Dasatinib
3. nilotinib
4. Bosutinib
5. Ponatinib

Allogeneic Stem Cell Transplant: For some patients, especially those with advanced CML or those who don't respond well to TKIs, this approach may be investigated. This means that the damaged bone marrow will be replaced with healthy stem cells from a compatible donor.

Clinical Trials: Participating in clinical trials can lead to the development of novel medicines and the ongoing advancement of CML research. These trials look at new drugs or drug combinations to expand treatment choices.

Monitoring and Adjusting Therapy: Regular monitoring using blood tests and other diagnostic methods helps assess the effectiveness of a treatment. The course of treatment may need to be changed in response to the patient's response and any side effects.

Supportive Care: Controlling symptoms and side effects is a crucial part of treating CML. Examples of supportive care interventions include receiving blood transfusions, attending to other medical conditions, and managing the negative effects of prescribed medications.

Combination Therapies: In certain cases, combining different TKIs or taking additional drugs into account may be considered to increase the effectiveness of therapy.

Treatment-Free Remission (TFR): A small number of patients may now be able to quit taking their medication while under strict observation if they have reacted significantly and sustainably to TKI therapy. This approach of remission without therapy is being studied in clinical trials.

The prognosis for those with CML has improved with the development of TKIs, and many can now have happy, fulfilled lives. Options for treatment are very individualized and depend on the patient's overall health, response to therapy, and illness stage. Following the treatment plan and keeping in constant contact with medical professionals are essential for the successful long-term management of CML.

Motives and Risk Factors

Leukemia is a complex group of blood cancers for which the exact causes are still unknown. Nonetheless, a variety of risk factors have been identified, and leukemia may develop as a result of certain illnesses. Here's a summary:

Reasons

Genetic Mutations: Changes to the DNA of blood cells can lead to uncontrolled cell division, which contributes to the development of leukemia. Specific genetic changes, such as those affecting the Philadelphia chromosome in Chronic Myeloid Leukemia (CML), have been related to specific types of leukemia.

Exposure to the Environment: Prolonged exposure to certain environmental factors has been linked to an increased risk of leukemia. Among these include ionizing radiation and benzene. This is particularly common in workplace settings where employees may be subjected to these chemicals.

CHAPTER FIVE

Genetic Factors: There is a chance that leukemia is related to genetic predispositions. Individuals with a slight elevated risk could include those with a family history of leukemia.

Dangerous Components

Age: While leukemia can affect anyone at any age, certain age groups are more likely to experience certain types of the disease. Acute lymphoblastic leukemia (ALL) is more prevalent in children, but chronic lymphocytic leukemia (CLL) is more common in older adults.

Gender: Some leukemia kinds have a little preference based on gender. For example, CLL is more common in men, although ALL is somewhat more common in boys throughout childhood but more common in girls during adulthood.

Previous Cancer Treatment: Individuals who have undergone radiation therapy or chemotherapy, for instance, may be at a higher risk of developing leukemia in the future.

Certain genetic abnormalities: Certain genetic abnormalities, like Down syndrome, have been linked to an increased risk of leukemia.

Family History: Despite the fact that most leukemia cases are uncommon, having a close family with the illness may slightly raise your risk.

Specific Blood Abnormalities: Individuals with certain blood abnormalities, such as myelodysplastic syndromes (MDS), are at a higher risk of developing leukemia.

It's important to keep in mind that having one or more risk factors does not guarantee that leukemia will develop; in fact, a large percentage of people who receive a leukemia diagnosis do not have any recognized risk factors. In addition, leukemia is a diverse set of illnesses with a range of risk factors linked to distinct subtypes. Regular medical exams and awareness of potential symptoms can help with early discovery and treatment.

Leukemia is a general term for blood cancers that can present with a wide range of symptoms. The specific symptoms and diagnosis techniques may vary depending on the type of leukemia. Here's a general synopsis:

Symptoms of leukemia include:

fatigue: Persistent, inexplicable exhaustion is one of the most common symptoms. Leukemia cells may push out normal blood cells in the bone marrow, resulting in a decrease in healthy blood cells.

Often Occurring Infections: Leukemia cells have the ability to compromise immune system performance, rendering an individual more susceptible to infections.

Easy Bleeding or Bruising: Leukemia can interfere with the body's normal platelet synthesis, resulting in bleeding gums, nosebleeds, or easy bruising.

Unexplained Weight Loss: Leukemia's impact on the body's metabolism may result in unexpectedly quick weight loss.

Joint and Bone Pain: Acute leukemia patients are more prone to feel pain in their joints and bones.

Increased Liver, Spleen, or Lymph Nodes: It is more typical for leukemia to cause palpable or visible enlargements in these organs.

Night Sweats: Regardless of the room's temperature or external factors, excessive perspiration might occur at night.

Liver or splenic enlargement may cause discomfort or a feeling of fullness in the abdomen.

Leukemia identification:

Blood Tests: A complete blood count (CBC) is often performed as the initial diagnostic test. If platelet, red blood cell, or white blood cell counts are abnormal, leukemia may be considered.

Bone Marrow Aspiration and Biopsy: A small sample of bone marrow is extracted from the hip bone using a needle. Under a microscope, the sample is examined to determine the kind and presence of leukemia cells.

Cytogenetic analysis: This technique looks for specific genetic abnormalities in the diseased cells' chromosomes to help identify the kind of leukemia.

Immunophenotyping: This method helps determine the kind of leukemia by examining the proteins on the surface of cells.

Imaging studies: X-rays, CT scans, or MRIs may be carried out to ascertain whether leukemia cells have spread to other organs or tissues.

Lumbar Puncture (Spinal Tap): Under some conditions, a lumbar puncture may be required to obtain a sample of cerebrospinal fluid from the spinal canal. This makes it easier to determine whether the central nervous system has been colonized by leukemia cells.

Early and accurate diagnosis is crucial for the development of a treatment plan that is appropriate for the specific kind and characteristics of leukemia and for the fast start of therapies. A person should see a doctor for a thorough evaluation when symptoms worsen or become persistent.

Treatment Options

Treatment for leukemia is primarily determined by the specific type of leukemia, its subtype, the patient's overall health, and other personal factors. Here are some common therapeutic options:

1. Chemotherapy:

Overview: The purpose of chemotherapy is to use drugs to destroy cancer cells in order to limit their proliferation.

Administration: It can be taken orally or administered by injection into the bloodstream.

Combination Therapies: A variety of chemotherapy drugs are commonly used in tandem to maximize efficacy.

2. Personalized Health Care:

Overview: Targeted therapies concentrate on particular substances or pathways that contribute to the growth of cancer cells.

For Chronic Myeloid Leukemia (CML), examples of targeted therapy include nilotinib, dasatinib, and imatinib.

3. Immunotherapy:

Overview: Immunotherapy aids the body in identifying and getting rid of cancer cells by boosting the immune system.

Monoclonal Antibodies: Rituximab and alemtuzumab are two common drugs used to treat leukemia.

4. Transfer of Allogeneic Stem Cells:

Overview: In this technique, sick or damaged bone marrow is replaced with healthy stem cells from a compatible donor.

Indications: Allogeneic stem cell transplantation is often considered for certain kinds of leukemia in circumstances of high-risk leukemia or relapse.

5. Radiation Therapy:

Overview: In radiation therapy, high-energy beams are utilized to target and destroy cancer cells.

Indications: It is commonly used to treat leukemia that has spread to the central nervous system or other body areas.

6. Hormone Treatment:

Overview: Hormone therapy is a treatment option for some types of leukemia that aims to stop the synthesis or activity of hormones that promote the growth of cancer.

7. Clinical Examinations:

Overview: Taking part in clinical trials advances leukemia research and gives people access to experimental therapies.

Novel Therapies: Clinical trials are frequently used to explore novel medicine combinations or experimental medications.

8. Assistive Healthcare:

Overview: The goals of supportive care include symptom management, averting complications, and enhancing the patient's general health.

Blood Transfusions: Transfusions may be given to people who have low blood cell counts.

9. Cautious Awaiting

Overview: In some circumstances, a watch-and-wait strategy with routine monitoring may be used, particularly for indolent or early-stage leukemia.

10. Remission without treatment (TFR):

Overview: Patients who experience a profound and long-lasting response to therapy may occasionally be able to stop taking it while being closely monitored.

Together with their healthcare team, the patient and they decide on a course of treatment, taking into account the patient's preferences, general health, and the unique features of their leukemia. Research continues to yield novel and focused therapy choices, hence improving leukemia patients' prognoses.

Having Leukemia

Navigating a unique road that blends medical management, emotional fortitude, and an emphasis on general well-being is what it means to have leukemia. Here are some things to think about:

1. Medical Supervision:

Frequent Monitoring: To evaluate the response to treatment and handle any possible adverse effects, leukemia frequently has to be monitored medically on a regular basis.

Treatment Adherence: Following the recommended course of action is essential for the successful management of the illness, regardless of whether it calls for chemotherapy, targeted therapy, or other modalities.

2. Emotional Health:

Support Systems: Establishing a robust network of family, friends, and medical professionals can help with both practical and emotional support.

Therapy and Counseling: Individual or group therapy can assist people in overcoming the psychological difficulties associated with having leukemia.

CHAPTER SIX

3. A Look at Lifestyle:

Healthy Lifestyle: Including regular exercise, a balanced diet, and enough sleep in your lifestyle can help you feel better overall.

Stress management: You can manage stress by using practices like mindfulness, meditation, and relaxation.

4. Interaction:

Open Communication: It's critical to communicate well with healthcare professionals. Talk about any worries, signs, or adverse consequences right away.

Educating Family and Friends: Giving loved ones with leukemia knowledge makes it easier for them to comprehend the difficulties and offer helpful assistance.

5. Self-Helding:

Listen to Your Body: Be aware of the cues your body sends you, and let your healthcare provider know if anything changes.

Taking Breaks: Making self-care a priority and taking breaks are acceptable. It's critical to strike a balance between work and rest.

6. Participation in the Community:

Connecting with Others: People with leukemia can make connections with others going through similar struggles by joining support groups or internet forums.

Advocacy: Some people make the decision to take on the role of advocate, spreading knowledge about leukemia and taking part in campaigns to fund medical research and other projects.

7. Long-Term Things to Think About:

Follow-Up Care: To keep an eye out for any indications of recurrence, even after reaching remission, routine follow-up visits are crucial.

Considering the Future: Talking with loved ones and healthcare professionals about long-term goals and preferences might give you a sense of control.

8. Remission without treatment (TFR):

Possibilities for TFR: Patients may, under some circumstances, talk to their medical team about the prospect of treatment-free remission. This entails stopping medication while under constant observation.

Leukemia living is a complex journey that calls for an all-encompassing strategy. A higher quality of life is a result of interacting with healthcare professionals, looking for emotional support, and adopting healthy lifestyle choices. It is critical that people with leukemia speak up for themselves and take an active role in their care in order to build resilience and a sense of empowerment.

CONCLUSION

For individuals afflicted, leukemia, a varied group of blood malignancies, is a difficult and complex journey. Leukemia has witnessed tremendous breakthroughs in treatment options, which have improved outcomes and quality of life for many people, even though it still requires careful medical supervision. To sum up, consider these important points:

Improvements in Medical Care:

Targeted Therapies: The advent of immunotherapies and tyrosine kinase inhibitors (TKIs) has completely changed the treatment paradigm by offering safer, more potent substitutes for conventional chemotherapy.

Higher Survival Rates: Better long-term results and higher survival rates have been attained by improvements in supportive care, early identification, and customized treatment regimens.

Treatment-Free Remission (TFR): This illustrates the dynamic nature of leukemia care, some patients, particularly those with specific forms of leukemia, may be eligible for treatment-free remission.

All-encompassing Care:

Emotional assistance: Because leukemia has an emotional toll, medical professionals are emphasizing more and more the value of psychological assistance and counseling for patients and their families.

Patient empowerment is encouraging patients to express their choices, take an active role in their care, and stand up for their own health.

Continuous Difficulties:

Variety of Leukemia Types: Due to the heterogeneous nature of leukemia, each case must be treated uniquely, taking into account the patient's genetic makeup, general health, and kind of leukemia.

Long-Term Monitoring: To identify any early indicators of recurrence, routine monitoring and follow-up care are still essential even after reaching remission.

Hope and Investigations:

Current Research: Through clinical trials, the field of leukemia research is still investigating novel medicines, focused therapy, and creative strategies.

Improvements in Knowledge: Accurate diagnosis and individualized treatment plans are made possible by growing knowledge of the genetic and molecular causes of leukemia.

Customized Tours:

Diverse Patient Experiences: Every person's experience with leukemia is different, and elements including age, general health, and reaction to treatment influence the journey.

Patient Support Communities: The formation of advocacy groups and patient support communities has produced forums for the exchange of knowledge, resources, and firsthand accounts.

In conclusion, even though leukemia presents many difficulties, advancements in research, patient care, and medical technology give hope and the possibility of a more resilient and manageable journey for people who have the disease. The future of leukemia treatment will be greatly influenced by ongoing efforts in research, patient care, and awareness.

THE END